ANDRE MOREIRA CASTILHO
HENRIQUE ELIAS DARMSTADTER
PEDRO AUGUSTO ROCHA TORRES

Idiopathic Scoliosis Screening

ANDRE MOREIRA CASTILHO
HENRIQUE ELIAS DARMSTADTER
PEDRO AUGUSTO ROCHA TORRES

Idiopathic Scoliosis Screening

ScienciaScripts

Cover image: www.ingimage.com

This book is a translation from the original published under ISBN 978-620-5-50413-0.

Publisher:
Sciencia Scripts
is a trademark of
Dodo Books Indian Ocean Ltd. and OmniScriptum S.R.L publishing group

120 High Road, East Finchley, London, N2 9ED, United Kingdom
Str. Armeneasca 28/1, office 1, Chisinau MD-2012, Republic of Moldova, Europe
Printed at: see last page
ISBN: 978-620-5-58490-3

Dedication

I dedicate to my wife, Ana Luiza, who always supported my endeavor and helped me throughout this important stage of my life. Thank you for your understanding, companionship, love, and especially for providing me with the structure and tranquility necessary to conclude this journey.

Thanks to

To my mentor, Dr. Asdrúbal, for his excellence and patience to teach. Not limiting himself only in helping with my thesis, but inserting me in the world of research and providing me to participate in events in the AOSpine community, in national and international scientific production. A period of building great admiration, respect, and gratitude. I hope to continue the path and honor my learning.

To my fellow master's students, André Arruda and Vitor Bonan. Two years in which we created a friendship that I will carry with me for life. Without your help, stimulus, and competence my path would be poorer and more difficult.

To my classmates. As a "foreigner", you welcomed me, helped me and introduced me to Caxias do Sul, a city that today I have a very special affection for.

To my residents, Pedro, Haroldo, and Angelo who worked hard on the data collection and helped in the writing of the paper. It would not have been possible to complete without your help.

To Kamila, my co-worker, for her dedication and great efficiency in organizing the data collection at the school, talking to principals and employees, ensuring the correct collection of the terms with great care so that everything happened in the most correct way possible. Thank you for your perfectionism and availability to make this project possible.

To the employees of the Marconi municipal school and of Club Olympico, thank you for helping to structure the collection by making the space available, organizing the groups, and understanding the project's objective. To the parents and students for making our project possible.

To my family for always supporting my choices and rooting for the completion of my dreams.

Summary

1 INTRODUCTION

Scoliosis is a pathology of the spine prevalent among children, adolescents, and young adults(1, 2). Scoliosis affects about 1% to 13.8% of children and adolescents(1, 2, 5, 6). There is a reasonably higher incidence among girls than boys, especially when it comes to more pronounced curvatures, emphasizing that girls are more susceptible to curvature progression(1, 5-9).

Scoliosis is defined as a lateral curvature of the spine equal to or greater than 10° (ten degrees), diagnosed by simple radiographic examination(1, 2, 10-12). Typically, patients with scoliosis have ample thoracic and limb functional capacity(13). However, late diagnosis cases that present curvature progression may present cardiopulmonary complications due to the rib cage deformity(1, 2,14). O treatment of patients with scoliosis ranges from observation, use of a brace, and surgery, and the prognosis is related to the degree of curvature(1, 2, 11). Therefore, early diagnosis is essential to guide treatment and prevent progression of the curvature.

The main findings of scoliosis on physical examination are asymmetry of the shoulders, scapulae, waist, trunk, and ribs(1). The Adams test evaluates the presence of gibbus and quantifies the lateral curvature, and is considered fundamental for scoliosis screening in schools(2, 5, 6).

Because of the especially high prevalence among children and adolescents, scoliosis screening has been widely performed in schools, providing an increase in the effectiveness of treatment and prevention measures(14-16). A study conducted in Hong Kong showed that the total cost of screening, diagnosis, and follow-up-about $3 million-is easily offset if at least 152 children receive conservative treatment that eliminates the need for surgery(17). The work published by a research group from the University of Caxias do Sul, pointed out that spine surgeries represented an expense for the Unified Health System (SUS) in 2014 of R$146,500,000.00, without considering expenses with non-operative care, diagnostic procedures, and costs related to loss of productivity and disability (18).

The screening policy has been widely debated, and several are the criticisms related to its cost-effectiveness, as well as to the number of referrals and unnecessary additional tests(5, 9, 15). Still, early diagnosis is crucial for reducing scoliosis-related morbidities.

The objective of this study is to verify the parameters of greater interobserver correlation of the various variables of the physical examination of idiopathic scoliosis with the aid of an application developed for a *smartphone*. Our study will serve as a basis for the future validation of the application as an effective tool in the treatment of idiopathic scoliosis.

2 REFERENCES

1. Hresko MT. Clinical practice. Idiopathic scoliosis in adolescents. N Engl J Med. 2013;368(9):834-41.
2. Weinstein SL, Dolan LA, Cheng JC, Danielsson A, Morcuende JA. Adolescent idiopathic scoliosis. Lancet. 2008;371(9623):1527-37.
3. Dunn J, Henrikson NB, Morrison CC, Nguyen M, Blasi PR, Lin JS. U.S. Preventive Services Task Force Evidence Syntheses, formerly Systematic Evidence Reviews. Screening for Adolescent Idiopathic Scoliosis: A Systematic Evidence Review for the US Preventive Services Task Force. Rockville (MD): Agency for Healthcare Research and Quality (US); 2018. 4. fong DY, Lee CF, Cheung KM, Cheng JC, Ng BK, Lam TP, et al. A meta-analysis of the clinical effectiveness of school scoliosis screening. Spine (Phila Pa 1976). 2010;35(10):106171.
5. Horne JP, Flannery R, Usman S. Adolescent idiopathic scoliosis: diagnosis and management. American family physician. 2014;89(3):193-8.
6. Grauers A, Einarsdottir E, Gerdhem P. Genetics and pathogenesis of idiopathic scoliosis. Scoliosis and spinal disorders. 2016;11:45.
7. Tan KJ, Moe MM, Vaithinathan R, Wong HK. Curve progression in idiopathic scoliosis: follow-up study to skeletal maturity. Spine. 2009;34(7):697- 700.
8. Lonstein JE, Carlson JM. The prediction of curve progression in untreated idiopathic scoliosis during growth. The Journal of bone and joint surgery American volume.
1984;66(7):1061-71.
9. Luk KD, Lee CF, Cheung KM, Cheng JC, Ng BK, Lam TP, et al. Clinical effectiveness of school screening for adolescent idiopathic scoliosis: a large population-based retrospective cohort study. Spine. 2010;35(17):1607-14.
10. Schwab F, el-Fegoun AB, Gamez L, Goodman H, Farcy JP. A lumbar classification of scoliosis in the adult patient: preliminary approach. Spine. 2005;30(14):1670-3. 11. Shaw R, Skovrlj B, Cho SK. Association Between Age and Complications in Adult Scoliosis Surgery: An Analysis of the Scoliosis Research Society Morbidity and Mortality Database. Spine. 2016;41(6):508-14.
12. Kim H, Kim HS, Moon ES, Yoon CS, Chung TS, Song HT, et al. Scoliosis imaging: what radiologists should know. Radiographics : a review publication of the Radiological Society of North America, Inc. 2010;30(7):1823-42.
13. Weinstein SL, Dolan LA, Spratt KF, Peterson KK, Spoonamore MJ, Ponseti IV. Health and function of patients with untreated idiopathic scoliosis: a 50-year natural history study.
Jama. 2003;289(5):559-67.

14. Zhang H, Guo C, Tang M, Liu S, Li J, Guo Q, et al. Prevalence of scoliosis among primary and middle school students in Mainland China: a systematic review and metaanalysis. Spine. 2015;40(1):41-9.
15. Suh SW, Modi HN, Yang JH, Hong JY. Idiopathic scoliosis in Korean schoolchildren: a prospective screening study of over 1 million children. European spine journal : official publication of the European Spine Society, the European Spinal Deformity Society, and the European Section of the Cervical Spine Research Society. 2011;20(7):1087-94.
16. de Souza FI, Di Ferreira RB, Labres D, Elias R, de Sousa AP, Pereira RE. Epidemiology of adolescent idiopathic scoliosis in students of the public schools in Goiania-GO. Acta Ortop Bras. 2013;21(4):223-5.
17. Lee CF, Fong DY, Cheung KM, Cheng JC, Ng BK, Lam TP, et al. Costs of school scoliosis screening: a large, population-based study. Spine (Phila Pa 1976). 2010;35(26):2266-72. 18. Teles AR, Righesso O, Gullo MC, Ghogawala Z, Falavigna A. Perspective of ValueBased Management of Spinal Disorders in Brazil. World neurosurgery. 2016;87:346-54.
19. Franko OI, Bray C, Newton PO. Validation of a scoliometer smartphone app to assess scoliosis. J Pediatr Orthop. 2012;32(8):e72-5.
20. Izatt MT, Bateman GR, Adam CJ. Evaluation of the iPhone with an acrylic sleeve versus the Scoliometer for rib hump measurement in scoliosis. Scoliosis. 2012;7(1):14. 21. Balg F, Juteau M, Theoret C, Svotelis A, Grenier G. Validity and reliability of the iPhone to measure rib hump in scoliosis. J Pediatr Orthop. 2014;34(8):774-9.
22. Driscoll M, Fortier-Tougas C, Labelle H, Parent S, Mac-Thiong JM. Evaluation of an apparatus to be combined with a smartphone for the early detection of spinal deformities.
Scoliosis. 2014;9:10.
23. Naziri Q, Detolla J, Hayes W, Burekhovich S, Merola A, Akamnanu C, et al. A Systematic Review of All Smart Phone Applications Specifically Aimed for Use as a Scoliosis Screening Tool. J Long Term Eff Med Implants. 2018;28(1):25-30.
24. Linker B. A dangerous curve: the role of history in America's scoliosis screening programs. Am J Public Health. 2012;102(4):606-16.
25. Screening for Adolescent Idiopathic Scoliosis: Recommendation Statement. Am Fam Physician. 2018;97(10):Online.
26. Beausejour M, Goulet L, Parent S, Feldman DE, Turgeon I, Roy-Beaudry M, et al. The effectiveness of scoliosis screening programs: methods for systematic review and expert panel recommendations formulation. Scoliosis. 2013;8(1):12.
27. Labelle H, Richards SB, De Kleuver M, Grivas TB, Luk KD, Wong HK, et

al. Screening for adolescent idiopathic scoliosis: an information statement by the scoliosis research society international task force. Scoliosis. 2013;8:17.

28. Amendt LE, Ause-Ellias KL, Eybers JL, Wadsworth CT, Nielsen DH, Weinstein SL.

Validity and Reliability Testing of the Scoliometer®. Physical Therapy. 1990;70(2):108-17.

3 ARTICLE

Medicine

Interobserver findings in the validation process of a Smartphone Application as a Tool for Screening patients with scoliosis

--Manuscript Draft-

Manuscript Number:	
Article Type:	OA Quality Improvement Study (SQUIRE Compliant)
Section/Category:	6600 Public health
Keywords:	scoliosis; idiopathic scoliosis; scoliosis screening; smartphone application; Spine; Spine surgery
Corresponding Author:	PEDRO AUGUSTO ROCHA TORRES, M.D. Hospital Madre Teresa BELO HORIZONTE, MINAS GERAIS BRAZIL
First Author:	ANDRE MOREIRA CASTILHO, M.D. Orthopedist, Spine Surgeon
Order of Authors:	ANDRE MOREIRA CASTILHO, M.D. Orthopedist, Spine Surgeon
	PEDRO AUGUSTO ROCHA TORRES, M.D. Orthopedist
	Kamila Rayane Campos Lopes, Biomedic, nursing technician
	Leonardo Pellizzoni, Information system specialist
	Orlando Righesso, M.D. Orthopedist, Spine Surgeon
	Asdrubal Falavigna, M.D. Neurosurgeon
Manuscript Region of Origin:	BRAZIL
Abstract:	Background : Scoliosis is a spinal condition that is common among children, adolescents, and young adults, affecting approximately 1%–13% of children and adolescents worldwide. Early diagnosis of scoliosis allows treatment in its initial stages and avoids surgical treatment and deformity progression. The present study aims to analyze the best correlated clinical parameters among examiners using an application for smartphone developed for screening of idiopathic scoliosis and to evaluate the friendly use of this application. Methods : This study assesses a smartphone mobile application that analyzes several clinical parameters related to the changes observed in scoliosis. Comparative analyses between medical and non-medical examiners were performed to define parameters with the greatest inter-observer correlation. Results : 89 participants have been examined, 18 were women and 71 were men. Two subjects were excluded from the analysis. The mean age of subjects from the public school was 11.30 years and from the sports club was 11.92 years. None of the parameters between examiners achieved perfect concordance. Substantial concordance was noted in reduced lordosis and mid-thoracic scoliometer. Moderate concordance was noted in pelvic asymmetry (frontal). Fair agreement was achieved in increased kyphosis, presence of a hump (frontal), waist asymmetry (frontal), ribcage asymmetry (frontal) and pelvic asymmetry (frontal). Conclusions : Screening for idiopathic scoliosis is a public health concern. The search for a tool that is inexpensive and technically and clinically effective is the final objective of our research. This is a preliminary study that will help to achieve our final goal that is the validation of an effective tool that can be used by nonmedical professional in the idiopathic scoliosis screening. Level of Evidence: III

Interobserver Findings in the Process of Validating a Smartphone Application as a Tool for Screening Scoliosis Patients

Castilho AM1; Torres PAR[2] ; Campos K3; Pellizzoni L[1] ; Righesso O[1] ;

Falavigna A[1]

1 Graduate Program in Health Sciences at the University of Caxias do Sul (UCS)

2 Orthopedist Specializing in Spine Surgery at Hospital Madre Teresa (HMT)

3 Biomedical nurse technician

Summary

Introduction: Scoliosis is a spinal condition that is common among children, adolescents and young adults, affecting approximately 1% to 13% of children and adolescents worldwide. Early diagnosis of scoliosis allows treatment in its early stages and avoids surgical treatment and progression of the deformity. The present study aims to analyze the most correlated clinical parameters among examiners using a smartphone application developed for idiopathic scoliosis screening and to evaluate the user friendliness of this application.

Methods: This study evaluates a mobile smartphone application that analyzes several clinical parameters related to the changes observed in scoliosis. Comparative analyses between medical and non-medical examiners were performed to define parameters with the highest interobserver correlation.

Results: 89 participants were examined, 18 were female and 71 were male. Two subjects were excluded from the analysis. The mean age of the subjects from the public school was 11.30 years and from the sports club was 11.92 years. None of the parameters between the examiners obtained perfect agreement. Substantial agreement was observed in reduced lordosis and scoliometer mean tothoracic assessment. Moderate agreement was observed in pelvic (frontal) asymmetry. Little agreement was reached in increased kyphosis, presence of giba (frontal), waist asymmetry (frontal), rib cage asymmetry (frontal), and pelvic asymmetry (frontal).

Conclusions: Screening for idiopathic scoliosis is a public health issue. The search for a tool that is inexpensive and technically and clinically effective is the ultimate goal of our research. This is a preliminary study that will help achieve our ultimate goal which is the validation of an effective tool that can be used by non-medical professionals in screening for idiopathic scoliosis.

Level of evidence: III

Abstract

Background: Scoliosis is a spinal condition that is common among children, adolescents, and young adults, affecting approximately 1%-13% of children and adolescents worldwide. Early diagnosis of scoliosis allows treatment in its initial stages and avoids surgical treatment and deformity progression. The present study aims to analyze the best correlated clinical parameters among examiners using an application for smartphone developed for screening of idiopathic scoliosis and to evaluate the friendly use of this application.

Methods: This study assesses a smartphone mobile application that analyzes several clinical parameters related to the changes observed in scoliosis. Comparative analyses between medical and non-medical examiners were performed to define parameters with the greatest interobserver correlation.

Results: 89 participants have been examined, 18 were women and 71 were men. Two subjects were excluded from the analysis. The mean age of subjects from the public school was 11.30 years and from the sports club was 11.92 years. None of the parameters between examiners achieved perfect concordance. Substantial concordance was noted in reduced lordosis and mid-thoracic scoliometer. Moderate concordance was noted in pelvic asymmetry (frontal). Fair agreement was achieved in increased kyphosis, presence of a hump (frontal), waist asymmetry (frontal), ribcage asymmetry (frontal) and pelvic asymmetry (frontal).

Conclusions: Screening for idiopathic scoliosis is a public health concern. The search for a tool that is inexpensive and technically and clinically effective is the final objective of our research. This is a preliminary study that will help to achieve our final goal that is the validation of an effective tool that can be used by nonmedical professional in the idiopathic scoliosis screening.

Level of Evidence: III

Introduction

Scoliosis is a spinal condition that is common among children, adolescents, and young adults.(1, 2) It affects approximately 1%-13% of children and adolescents worldwide.(1, 2, 5, 6) Most patients with scoliosis have a mild abnormal curvature of the spine and the curvature does not progress into adulthood. (2) However, more pronounced curvature and late diagnosis can lead to cardiopulmonary complications and reduced quality of life for patients.(1, 3) Early diagnosis of scoliosis allows timely treatment of the condition in its early stages, avoiding surgical treatment and progression of the deformity.(1) Screening for idiopathic scoliosis is widely discussed in the medical literature. (4) It has been performed in schools because of its high prevalence among children and adolescents, increasing the effectiveness of treatment and preventive measures and reducing the costs of surgery. (7-9) Major findings of scoliosis on physical examination are asymmetry of the shoulders, scapulae, pelvis, trunk, and rib cage. (1) The Adams forward bending test is used to assess the presence of a bulge and quantify lateral curvature; it is considered essential for scoliosis screening in schools. (2, 5, 6) The screening policy has been the subject of debate and there are several criticisms about the related cost/benefit ratio, number of referrals, and unnecessary complementary tests.(5, 7, 10) However, early diagnosis is still essential for reducing the morbidities associated with scoliosis. The present study aims to analyze the best clinical correlation of parameters between examiners using a smartphone application (app) developed for idiopathic scoliosis screening and to evaluate the user friendliness of this app.

Methods

Type of study

We conducted a cross-sectional study to evaluate idiopathic scoliosis in schoolchildren aged 8 to 17 years from a public school and a private school and an athletic club in Belo Horizonte, Minas Gerais, Brazil. The project was approved by the Ethics Committee of the Hospital Mater Dei in Belo Horizonte (Ethics Evaluation Submission Certificate - CAAE no. 07926919.5.0000.5128). Patient confidentiality and privacy will be guaranteed at all stages of the study, according to the principles of medical ethics.

Eligibility Criteria

Inclusion Criteria

1. Public school students, private school students, and athletes from a sports club in the city of Belo Horizonte who were between the ages of 8 to 17 years old, who voluntarily agreed to participate in the study and signed an informed consent document. The guardians of the participants also needed to sign an informed consent form.

Exclusion criteria

1. Previous spine surgery.
2. Diagnosis and early treatment of scoliosis.
3. Diseases of the nervous system that compromise ambulation.
4. Cognitive or comprehension problems.

Sample Size Calculation

The post hoc sample size calculation was done using R software using the cohen. kappa (irr) with a 5% agreement level and a 95% confidence interval. Considering all variables analyzed and in comparison with each examiner the average number of participants was 88 (minimum 56 and maximum 145).

Study Sites

The sites were selected based on those that were the most representative of the sample: a public school in the municipality of Belo Horizonte and a private sports club in Belo Horizonte. Data were first collected in the public school. Due to bureaucratic difficulties at the public school and also to have a more heterogeneous profile of the sample, we expanded the locations to a sports club and a private school. In these two locations we had a more controlled environment. In the sports club we started the research among boys, all basketball players, and before we could enroll the female group in the analysis, we had to interrupt our study because of the COVID 19 pandemic.

We also could not evaluate the private school students for the same reason.

Selecting and training examiners

The examiners were selected to include at least one examiner experienced in the assessment of individuals with adolescent idiopathic scoliosis (gold standard examiner), one orthopedic surgeon specializing in spine surgery (inexperienced medical examiner), and one non-medical examiner. The examiners were trained for this activity and supervised by the principal investigator specializing in scoliosis. The team of examiners consisted of an orthopedic specialist in spine surgery (ExL), a surgical instrumental nurse technician (Ex1), and an orthopedic surgeon in the first year of training in spine surgery (Ex2).

Application description

Children and adolescents were assessed by the "Scoliosis Screen mobile app", available for iOS or Android (see attachment: https://youtu.be/fs3aNbNf404). The app was developed at the University of Caxias do Sul and is available in the Brazilian Apple and Google Store. The evaluators were trained to use the software application and its tutorials.

Variables analyzed

The app evaluates the following variables: head, shoulder, waist, rib cage and pelvic asymmetry by anterior and posterior vision, the presence of kyphosis and a gyphosis (Adams test); and finally, the measurement of an upper, middle and lower thoracic scoliosis using the scoliometer (included in the evaluation sequence using the accelerometer of the Smartphone). The interobserver correlation of these variables between examiners and also the time spent on each assessment was measured and compared.

Phases of the evaluation

The examination of each individual was conducted by two alternating examiners as follows: - Ex1 - ExL; Ex1 - Ex2. The individuals wore a short-sleeved t-shirt and shorts or a shirt. The examination was conducted in a private, quiet environment. Subjects with a positive Adams test, shoulder asymmetry, and a scoliotometer reading of >2° were invited to participate in a free consultation with the principal investigator. These clinical criteria were chosen at this first time point to increase the sensitivity of the evaluation, designing a second evaluation with the lead examiner in an attempt to validate the application. The lead researcher receives an e-mail from the app whenever changes are detected and sends a letter to the guardians inviting them to a specialized medical consultation.

Application Evaluation

The examiners were asked to complete the Post Study System Usability Questionnaire (PSSUQ) (11, 12) to evaluate the software application. The survey consists of 19 items scored from 1 to 7, ranging from "strongly disagree" to "strongly agree". The items analyzed were ease, simplicity, effectiveness, ability to complete tasks quickly, ability to complete tasks, comfort, ease of learning, productivity possibility, system's ability to correct problems, ability to resolve errors, quality system information , information accessibility, information compression in the system, efficiency of system information, organization of system information, system interface, system interface satisfaction, system expectations, and overall satisfaction.

Statistical Analysis

The collected data were initially entered into an Excel spreadsheet (2013) and later analyzed in the statistical package SPSS (26.0). The normality of continuous data was assessed by the Shapiro-Wilk test. Anthropometric data were expressed as mean, standard deviation, median, and minimum value and maximum values. The examination time between the researcher and the examiner were compared using the Mann Whitney U-test. The changes observed in the physical examination were presented in contingency tables and expressed as absolute (n) and relative frequencies (%). The agreement between the researcher and the examiner was evaluated with the Kappa test. The significance level was set at 5% ($p < 0.05$) in all analyses.

Results

Anthropometric data

Data collection was conducted between the months of August and December 2019. The number of participants was 89. Of these, 18 were female and 71 were male. Two subjects were excluded from the analysis, namely, one subject who had already been diagnosed with neuromuscular scoliosis and one with adolescent idiopathic scoliosis under medical follow-up. The average age of the school public subjects was 11.3 years, average weight 39.0kg, average height 1.5 meters and average BMI (body mass index) 17.9 (table 1). The average age of the sports club was 11.92 years, average weight 61.2kg, average height 1.71 meters, and average BMI 20.3 (table 2).

Time Evaluation

The average time for subject examination was 57.18 seconds for ExL compared to 68.36 seconds for Ex1 (figure 1) and the average time for individual examination was 56.45 seconds for Ex1 compared to 56.25 seconds for Ex2 (figure 2).

Overall evaluation and interobserver correlations

ExL evaluated 54 subjects and referred 11 for reevaluation. Nine of them had shoulder asymmetry and two had curvature with a rotation >2°. Ex1 evaluated 87 individuals and referred 24 for reevaluation. Twenty-four of them had shoulder asymmetry, 5 had gibbousness, and 5 had changes in the scoliosometer readings. Ex2 evaluated 33 individuals and referred 11 of these, all with shoulder asymmetry. Tables 3 and 4 show the analysis of all variables and the positive correlations between the examiners. None of the parameters between ExL and Ex1 reached near perfect agreement. Substantial agreement was seen in reduced lordosis and change in mid-thoracic scoliotic measurement. Fair agreement was reached in increased kyphosis, presence of a giba (frontal) and waist asymmetry (frontal). All other parameters had mild or poor agreement. The presence of a giba, scapular asymmetry, and waist (posterior) asymmetry were statistically significant changes found between ExL and Ex1. In individuals diagnosed with asymmetrical shoulder, scapular (posterior), waist and pelvic (posterior and frontal) asymmetry, rib cage (frontal) asymmetry were found between ExL and Ex1 with statistical difference. None of the parameters between Ex1 and Ex2 reached near perfect and substantial agreement. Moderate agreement was observed in pelvic (frontal) asymmetry. Chest box (frontal) asymmetry and pelvic (frontal) asymmetry had reasonable agreement. In subjects diagnosed with shoulder, scapular (posterior), waist and pelvic (posterior and frontal) asymmetry, rib cage (frontal) had statistically significant agreement between Ex1 and Ex2.

Application Evaluation

The results of the application evaluation showed total user satisfaction in effectiveness, ease of learning, productive possibility, and satisfaction of the system interface. The worst scores in the evaluation were ease of use and troubleshooting ability on the part of the system and the user (table 5).

Discussion

This study is the first to evaluate almost all parameters of the physical examination between medical and non-medical examiners in an attempt to improve screening for adolescent idiopathic scoliosis. Our findings showed that reduced lordosis, altered scoliotometer measurement at mid-thorax, presence of giba, waist asymmetry, kyphosis, rib cage asymmetry, and pelvic asymmetry had fair agreement. Shoulder asymmetry, one of the parameters used as a warning in the app, showed poor interobserver correlation. The mean assessment time was initially significantly slower for the non-medical examiner (first group analysis), but improved considerably in the subsequent analysis (second group). This is probably because the non-medical examiner gained experience using the app. In addition, the interface of the app proved to be user-friendly. Adolescent idiopathic scoliosis is a common condition in the world population and has a high morbidity rate.(1), (3) Personal perception of poor health quality, poor self-image, and restricted social relationships are expected outcomes among patients whose deformities are maintained or progress through adulthood.(3) Failure to detect scoliosis at an early stage increases the risk of disease progression and severity.(13)

Screening for adolescent idiopathic scoliosis is a subject widely discussed in the literature.(4) The first screening program was implemented in 1962(14) in Delaware, USA, after Shands et al. at Alfred DuPont Hospital warned about the prevalence of idiopathic scoliosis in adolescents. In the following years, the number of US states joining the screening program increased, reaching over 20 states by 1989. (14) In 2004, the US in Preventive Service Task Force (USPFTS) advised against screening because of the high number of false positives, particularly in the Adams forward bending test.(15)

The Scoliosis Research Society (SRS), taking the USPFTS determination into consideration, initiated a study to determine the effectiveness of screening for adolescent idiopathic scoliosis. A group of experts was established to study the variables related to screening effectiveness.(16) Clinical and technical programs, costs, and treatment effectiveness were evaluated. After reviewing key questions in the medical literature, SRS screening recommendations were published in 2013.(17) The prevalence of adolescent idiopathic scoliosis, the proportion of patients referred for radiographic evaluation, and the positive predictive value are indicators of clinical effectiveness. A scoliometer is the best assessment tool, combined with or without the Adams forward bending test. Analysis of Moiré topography can increase the sensitivity and specificity of screening. The program recommends evaluation of girls aged 10 to 12 years and boys aged 13 to 14 years. Identifying patients in the early stages of the disease allows early treatment with the use of an orthopedic brace and reduces the risk of progression to severe deformities, thus indicating the effectiveness of the screening program. Evidence on cost-effectiveness in the literature is still insufficient.

The total cost of screening, diagnosis and monitoring - approximately three million dollars - can be easily offset if at least 152 children receive conservative treatment that eliminates the need for surgery (18). A study published by a research group at the University of Caxias do Sul indicated that in 2014, spine surgeries have a cost to Brazil's national health system - Sistema Único de Saúde (SUS) - of R$146.5 million, excluding expenses for surgical care, diagnostic procedures, and costs associated with lost productivity and disability (19) .

Numerous screening tools have been proposed for the detection of adolescent idiopathic scoliosis, of which measurement with a scoliometer is the most popular. (20) Several mobile apps have been validated after comparison with the scoliometer and become useful tools for in-office evaluation by specialists and in screening for adolescent idiopathic scoliosis. (21-24) Naziri et al. performed an evaluation of mobile scoliometers available in apps and concluded that the tools are at least as effective as the manual scoliometer, possibly more so, with no difference between paid and free apps.(25)

In recent years, the growth in smartphone use has revolutionized medical professionals' access to information. According to Franko et al. (21) 84% of orthopedic residents and nonphysician professionals on orthopedic teams use smartphones and 53% of them use mobile apps in clinical practice and that number is probably higher now. Most scoliosis screening apps use only the scoliometer as a measurement. Fong et al. demonstrated that screening performed using only the Adams forward bending test is insufficient and results in a high false positive rate.(4) The combination of the scoliometer, Adams forward bending test and Moiré topography has sensitivity and specificity close to 94% and 99%, respectively.(3) Our study presents a simplified alternative for the diagnosis and screening of adolescent idiopathic scoliosis. Most screening studies have been performed with the assistance of medical professionals, which implies a high health care cost.

The inclusion of various physical examination parameters of a patient with scoliosis will allow an evaluation of which parameters have the highest agreement, while outpatient evaluation by a spine specialist will allow validation of the application as a screening tool. In our initial results, reduced lordosis, altered scoliometer measurement at mid-thorax, and pelvic (frontal) asymmetry had better inter-examiner agreement.

These parameters need to be verified in the outpatient evaluation to be validated. This study had some limitations. The difficulty of data collection was one of the limitations of the study. It was also more difficult because of COVID 19. Because this is a screening study, our sample is not yet sufficiently representative, and another study will be needed for further evaluation and interpretation of the data. The application will require refinements to improve data storage and export. Time was measured by the examiners themselves, which represents a significant bias in the evaluation of this variable.

The quality of the comparative analysis will improve once we get the data from the paired comparison between the lead examiner and other non-medical examiners (considering that the data collected so far have been provided by only one non-medical examiner). It is also important to analyze the results of the physical examination and radiographs after referring individuals in whom the application showed changes to a specialist. We will then be able to validate the tool as a screening method. Interestingly, the time between medical and non-medical examiner was similar. There was a reduction for the non-medical examiner in the duration of the assessment comparing the first and second event.

Regarding future prospects, the main goal of the study is to create a simple and effective tool for screening adolescents with idiopathic scoliosis by non-medical professionals, especially in the school setting. This study has laid the foundation for the future creation of a simple and effective tool for idiopathic scoliosis screening. The final analysis of the data will allow adjustments to be made to the smartphone app that will ensure the ease of understanding and use of the tool and increase its sensitivity and specificity in detecting the disease. Improved cost-effectiveness will allow cities and states to diagnose and treat adolescent idiopathic scoliosis early. A more representative sample and a larger number of individuals and examiners will be needed to test the applicability of the tool. The results of the PSSUQ show that the application is user friendly in terms of simplicity, ease and effectiveness. It also shows that some modifications are needed to make it easier and more resolutive. Another possibility is to provide a simplified tutorial for users.

In conclusion, screening for idiopathic scoliosis is a public health issue. This is a preliminary study that will help achieve our ultimate goal, which is the validation of an effective tool that can be used by a non-medical professional to screen for idiopathic scoliosis.

References

1. Hresko MT. Clinical practice. Idiopathic scoliosis in adolescents. N Engl J Med. 2013;368(9):834-41.

2. Weinstein SL, Dolan LA, Cheng JC, Danielsson A, Morcuende JA. Adolescent idiopathic scoliosis. Lancet (London, England). 2008;371(9623):1527-37.

3. Dunn J, Henrikson NB, Morrison CC, Nguyen M, Blasi PR, Lin JS. U.S. Preventive Services Task Force Evidence Syntheses, formerly Systematic Evidence Reviews. Screening for Adolescent Idiopathic Scoliosis: A Systematic Evidence Review for the US Preventive Services Task Force. Rockville (MD): Agency for Healthcare Research and Quality (US); 2018. 4. fong DY, Lee CF, Cheung KM, Cheng JC, Ng BK, Lam TP, et al. A meta-analysis of the clinical effectiveness of school scoliosis screening. Spine (Phila Pa 1976). 2010;35(10):1061-71.

5. Horne JP, Flannery R, Usman S. Adolescent idiopathic scoliosis: diagnosis and management. American family physician. 2014;89(3):193-8.

6. Grauers A, Einarsdottir E, Gerdhem P. Genetics and pathogenesis of idiopathic scoliosis. Scoliosis and spinal disorders. 2016; 11:45.

7. Suh SW, Modi HN, Yang JH, Hong JY. Idiopathic scoliosis in Korean schoolchildren: a prospective screening study of over 1 million children.

   European spine journal: official publication of the European Spine Society, the European Spinal Deformity Society, and the European

Section of the Cervical Spine Research Society. 2011;20(7):1087-94.

8. de Souza FI, Di Ferreira RB, Labres D, Elias R, de Sousa AP, Pereira RE. Epidemiology of adolescent idiopathic scoliosis in students at the public schools in Goiania-GO. Acta ortopedica brasileira. 2013;21(4):223-5.

9. Zhang H, Guo C, Tang M, Liu S, Li J, Guo Q, et al. Prevalence of scoliosis among primary and middle school students in Mainland China: a systematic review and meta-analysis. Spine. 2015;40(1):41-9.

10. Luk KD, Lee CF, Cheung KM, Cheng JC, Ng BK, Lam TP, et al. Clinical effectiveness of school screening for adolescent idiopathic scoliosis: a large population-based retrospective cohort study. Spine. 2010;35(17):1607-14.

11. Rosa AF, Martins AI, Costa V, Queirós A, Silva A, Rocha NP, editors. European Portuguese validation of the post-study system usability questionnaire (PSSUQ). 2015 10th Iberian Conference on Information Systems and Technologies (CISTI); 2015: IEEE.

12. Lewis JR. Psychometric evaluation of the PSSUQ using data from five years of usability studies. International Journal of Human-Computer Interaction. 2002; 14(3-4):463-88.

13. Weinstein SL, Dolan LA, Spratt KF, Peterson KK, Spoonamore MJ, Ponseti IV. Health and function of patients with untreated idiopathic scoliosis: a 50-year natural history study. Jama. 2003;289(5):559-67.

14. Linker B. A dangerous curve: the role of history in America's scoliosis screening programs. Am J Public Health. 2012;102(4):606-16.

15. Screening for Adolescent Idiopathic Scoliosis: Recommendation

Statement. Am Fam Physician. 2018;97(10): Online.

16. Beauséjour M, Goulet L, Parent S, Feldman DE, Turgeon I, Roy-Beaudry M, et al. The effectiveness of scoliosis screening programs: methods for systematic review and expert panel recommendations formulation. Scoliosis. 2013;8(1):12.

17. Labelle H, Richards SB, De Kleuver M, Grivas TB, Luk KD, Wong HK, et al. Screening for adolescent idiopathic scoliosis: an information statement by the scoliosis research society international task force. Scoliosis. 2013; 8:17.

18. Hengwei F, Zifang H, Qifei W, Weiqing T, Nali D, Ping Y, et al. Prevalence of Idiopathic Scoliosis in Chinese Schoolchildren: A Large, Population-Based Study. Spine (Phila Pa 1976). 2016;41(3):259-64.

19. Teles AR, Righesso O, Gullo MC, Ghogawala Z, Falavigna A. Perspective of ValueBased Management of Spinal Disorders in Brazil. World neurosurgery. 2016; 87:346-54.

20. Amendt LE, Ause-Ellias KL, Eybers JL, Wadsworth CT, Nielsen DH, Weinstein SL. Validity and Reliability Testing of the Scoliometer®. Physical Therapy. 1990;70(2):108-17.

21. Franko OI, Bray C, Newton PO. Validation of a scoliometer smartphone app to assess scoliosis. J Pediatr Orthop. 2012;32(8): e72-5.

22. Izatt MT, Bateman GR, Adam CJ. Evaluation of the iPhone with an acrylic sleeve versus the Scoliometer for rib hump measurement in scoliosis. Scoliosis. 2012;7(1):14.

23. Balg F, Juteau M, Theoret C, Svotelis A, Grenier G. Validity and reliability of the iPhone to measure rib hump in scoliosis. J Pediatr Orthop. 2014;34(8):774-9.

24. Driscoll M, Fortier-Tougas C, Labelle H, Parent S, Mac-Thiong JM. Evaluation of an apparatus to be combined with a smartphone for the early detection of spinal deformities. Scoliosis. 2014; 9:10.

25. Naziri Q, Detolla J, Hayes W, Burekhovich S, Merola A, Akamnanu C, et al.

Systematic Review of All Smart Phone Applications Specifically Aimed for Use as a Scoliosis Screening Tool. J Long Term Eff Med Implants. 2018;28(1):25-30.

Figure legends

Figure 1. Boxplot comparing the assessment time between the examiners

*Mann-Whitney U-test

Figure 2: Boxplot comparing the assessment time between the examiners

*Mann-Whitney U-test

Table 1. Description of age and anthropometric profile of public school adolescents by different examiners

Table 2. Description of age and anthropometric profile of the adolescents of the sports club by different examiners

Table 3. Analysis of the agreement of changes in the physical examination between ExL and Ex1 examiners

Table 4. Analysis of the agreement of changes in the physical examination between Ex1 and Ex2 examiners

Table 5: Descriptive statistics of the examiners' evaluation.

Figure 1. Boxplot comparing the assessment time between the examiners

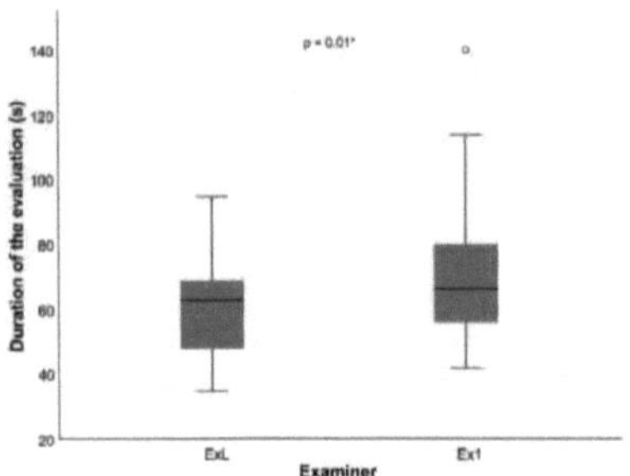

Figure 2: Boxplot comparing the assessment time between the examiners

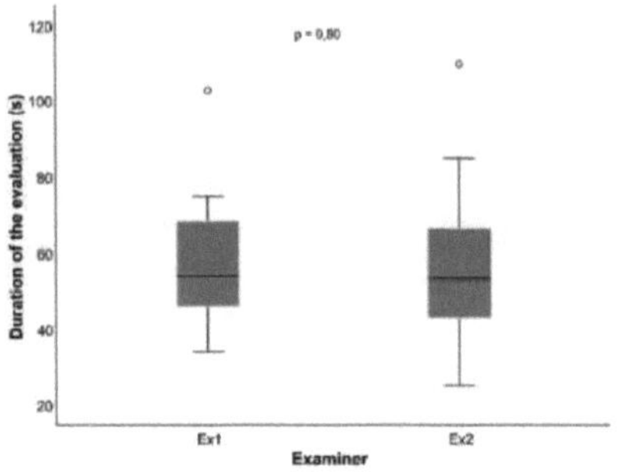

Table 1. Description of age and anthropometric profile of the adolescents from the public school by different examiners

	Mean	SD	Median	Minimum	Maximum
Age of the adolescent (years)	11.3	1.5	11.0	9.0	16.0
Weight (kg)	39.0	8.5	38.0	23.0	57.00
Height (cm)	150.0	10.0	152.0	130.0	163.0
BMI	17.9	2.2	17.5	14.3	21.6

SD, Standard deviation; BMI, Body Mass Index

Table 2. Description of age and anthropometric profile of the adolescents from sport club by different examiners

	Mean	SD	Median	Minimum	Maximum
Age of the adolescent (years)	11.9	1.4	12.0	8.0	14.0
Weight (kg)	61.2	19.1	56.0	34.0	99.0
Height (cm)	171.0	13.0	171.0	147.0	191.0
BMI	20.3	4.2	19.8	15.5	30.3

SD, Standard deviation; BMI, Body Mass Index

Table 3. Analysis of the agreement on the changes on physical examination between the examiners ExL and Ex1

	ExL n (%)	**Ex1 n (%)**	**Total**	***kappa***	***P***
Head asymmetry (Posterior)	0 (0.0)	0 (0.0)	0 (0.0)	na	na
Shoulder asymmetry (Posterior)	9 (16.7)	12 (22.2)	21 (19.4)	0.0	1.00
Scapular asymmetry (Posterior)	8 (14.8)	11 (20.4)	19 (17.6)	-0.08	0.54
Waist asymmetry (Posterior)	3 (5.6)	16 (29.6)	19 (17.6)	0.13	0.15
Pelvis asymmetry (Posterior)	4 (7.4)	13 (24.1)	17 (15.7)	0.14	0.20
Increased kyphosis	2 (3.7)	8 (14.8)	10 (9.3)	**0.36**	**0.01**
Reduced kyphosis	8 (14.8)	5 (9.3)	13 (12.0)	0.22	0.09
Increased lordosis	9 (16.7)	12 (22.2)	21 (19.4)	0.0	1.00
Reduced lordosis	3 (5.6)	2 (3.7)	5 (4.6)	**0.79**	**< 0.01**
Presence of a hump (Frontal)	2 (3.7)	4 (7.4)	6 (5.6)	**0.30**	**0.02**
Head asymmetry (Frontal)	1 (1.9)	0 (0.0)	1 (0.9)	na	na
Shoulder asymmetry (Frontal)	14 (25.9)	13 (24.1)	27 (25.0)	0.16	0.23
Ribcage asymmetry (Frontal)	4 (7.4)	4 (7.4)	8 (7.4)	0.19	0.16
Waist asymmetry (Frontal)	7 (13.0)	13 (24.1)	20 (18.5)	**0.29**	**0.03**
Pelvis asymmetry (Frontal)	5 (9.3)	14 (25.9)	19 (17.6)	0.08	0.45
Upper thoracic scoliometer	0 (0.0)	3 (5.6)	3 (2.8)	na	na
Mid-thoracic scoliometer	1 (1.9)	2 (3.7)	3 (2.8)	**0.66**	**< 0.01**
Lower thoracic scoliometer	1 (1.9)	3 (5.6)	4 (3.7)	- 0.03	0.80

ExL, examiner orthopedist specializing in spine surgery; n, absolute frequency; %, relative frequency; Ex1, examiner surgical instrument technician; *kappa*, Kappa test; na, not applicable

Table 4. Analysis of the agreement on the changes on physical examination between the examiners Ex1 and Ex2

	Ex1 n (%)	Ex2 n (%)	Total	*kappa*	*p*
Head asymmetry (Posterior)	0 (0.0)	1 (3.0)	1 (1.5)	0.00	1.00
Shoulder asymmetry (Posterior)	11 (33.3)	11 (33.3)	22 (33.3)	0.32	0.06
Scapular asymmetry (Posterior)	7 (21.2)	12 (36.4)	19 (28.8)	0.06	0.68
Waist asymmetry (Posterior)	8 (24.2)	9 (27.3)	17 (25.8)	0.29	0.09
Pelvic asymmetry (Posterior)	10 (30.3)	4 (12.1)	14 (21.2)	**0.31**	**0.03**
Increased kyphosis	9 (27.3)	3 (9.1)	12 (18.2)	0.03	0.80
Reduced kyphosis	1 (3.0)	1 (3.0)	2 (3.0)	−0.03	0.96
Increased lordosis	11 (33.3)	5 (15.2)	16 (24.2)	0.05	0.73
Reduced lordosis	1 (3.0)	2 (6.1)	3 (4.5)	−0.04	0.79
Presence of hump (Frontal)	1 (3.0)	0 (0.0)	1 (1.5)	0.00	1.00
Head asymmetry (Frontal)	0 (0.0)	1 (3.0)	1 (1.5)	0.00	1.00
Shoulder asymmetry (Frontal)	12 (36.4)	8 (24.2)	20 (30.3)	0.15	0.35
Ribcage asymmetry (Frontal)	4 (12.1)	10 (30.3)	14 (21.2)	**0.31**	**0.03**
Waist asymmetry (Frontal)	11 (33.3)	14 (42.4)	25 (37.9)	0.30	0.08
Pelvic asymmetry (Frontal)	13 (39.4)	11 (33.3)	24 (36.4)	**0.48**	**0.006**

Ex1, examiner surgical instrument technician; n, absolute frequency; %, relative frequency; Ex2 orthopedist in the first year of training in spine surgery; *kappa*, Kappa test; na, not applicable

Table 5. Description statistics of the examiners' evaluation.

	Mean	**SD**
Easiness	5.5	1.9
Simplicity	6.5	1.0
Effectiveness	7.0	0.0
Ability to complete tasks quickly	6.3	1.0
Ability to complete tasks	6.5	0.6
Comfort	6.5	1.0
Easiness to learn	7.0	0.0
Productivity possibility	7.0	0.0
System capacity to fix problems	5.5	1.0
Ability to solve mistakes	5.8	1.0
Quality system information	6.3	1.0
Accessibility to information	6.8	0.5
System infomation compreession	6.8	0.5
System information effectiveness	6.8	0.5
System infomation organization	6.5	1.0
System interface	7.0	0.0
System interface satisfaction	7.0	0.0
System expectations	6.5	1.0
System overall satisfaction	6.8	0.5

SD, Standard deviation

4 CONSIDERATIONS AND FUTURE PERSPECTIVES

The main objective of the work is to create a simple and efficient tool for the screening of adolescent idiopathic scoliosis by non-medical professionals, especially in a school environment. The analysis of the data will allow adjustments in the smartphone application that will guarantee the ease of understanding and application of the tool, as well as its greater sensitivity and specificity in the identification of the disease. The best cost-benefit ratio will allow municipalities and states the early diagnosis and treatment of adolescent idiopathic scoliosis. A more representative sample will be necessary, as well as a larger number of examiners to test the applicability of the tool.

Screening for adolescent idiopathic scoliosis is a public health concern. The search for a tool that is technically, clinically and cost-effective is the goal of our work. This preliminary study will define the basis for adjusting the developed smartphone application to find the expected result.

Application Images

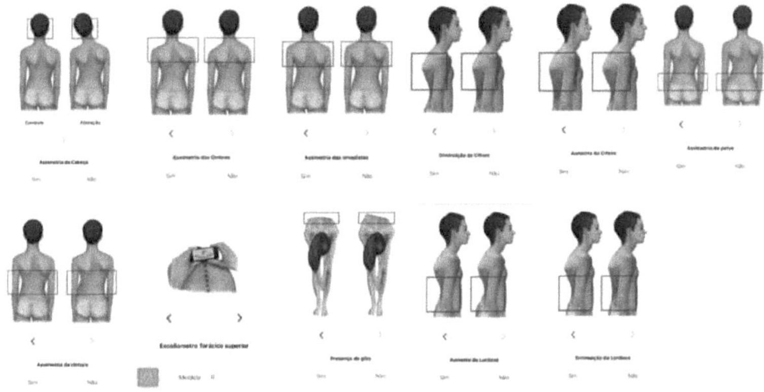

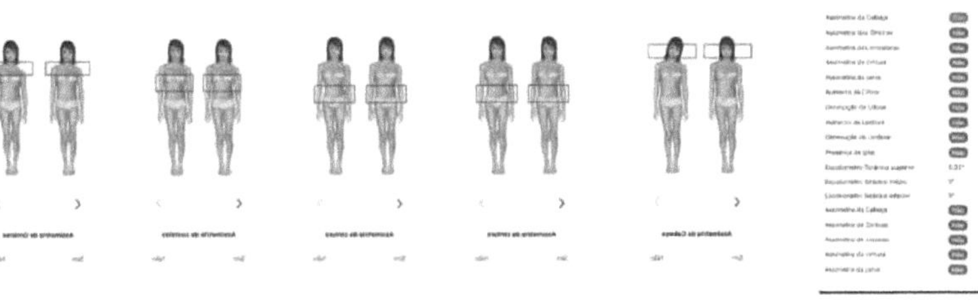

Applicability: PSSUQ

Perguntas	Muito insatisfeito------muito satisfeito						
No geral estou satisfeito com a facilidade de usar este sistema.	1	2	3	4	5	6	7
Foi simples de usar este sistema.	1	2	3	4	5	6	7
Eu poderia efetivamente completar as tarefas e cenários usando este sistema.	1	2	3	4	5	6	7
Consegui concluir as tarefas e cenários rapidamente usando este sistema.	1	2	3	4	5	6	7
Consegui concluir as tarefas e cenários eficientemente usando este sistema.	1	2	3	4	5	6	7
Eu me senti confortável usando este sistema.	1	2	3	4	5	6	7
Foi fácil aprender a usar este sistema.	1	2	3	4	5	6	7
Acredito que posso me tornar produtivo rapidamente usando este sistema.	1	2	3	4	5	6	7
O sistema deu mensagem de erro que me disseram claramente como corrigir os problemas.	1	2	3	4	5	6	7
Sempre que cometi um erro ao usar o sistema, eu consegui me recuperar com facilidade e rapidez.	1	2	3	4	5	6	7
As informações (como ajuda on-line, mensagens na tela e outras documentações) fornecidas com este sistema eram claras.	1	2	3	4	5	6	7
Foi fácil encontrar as informações que eu precisava.	1	2	3	4	5	6	7
As informações para o sistema eram fáceis de entender.	1	2	3	4	5	6	7
As informações foram eficazes e me ajudaram a completar as tarefas e cenários.	1	2	3	4	5	6	7
A organização das informações nas telas do sistema foi clara.	1	2	3	4	5	6	7
A interface deste sistema foi agradável.	1	2	3	4	5	6	7
Eu gostei de usar a interface deste sistema.	1	2	3	4	5	6	7
Este sistema tem todas as funções e capacidades que eu espero que ele tenha.	1	2	3	4	5	6	7
No geral estou satisfeito com este sistema.	1	2	3	4	5	6	7

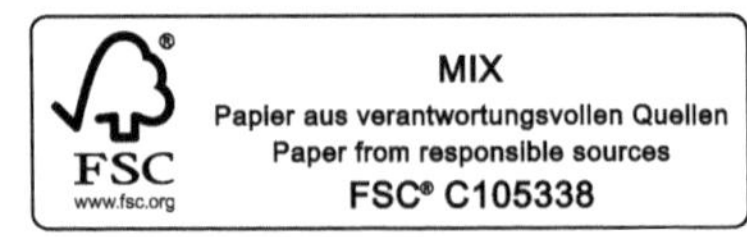

Printed by Books on Demand GmbH, Norderstedt / Germany